nF421186

## Table of Contents

# INTRODUCTION

There is nothing extraordinary about the Pritikin Diet aside from that it is incredibly solid. In excess of 100 investigations distributed in peer-inspected clinical diaries, the Pritikin Program of Diet and Exercise has been found to advance weight reduction as well as forestall and control a large number of the world's driving executioners, including diabetes, hypertension, and coronary illness.

While a great deal of the current weight control plans are regularly founded on the low measure of sugars, and the medium-high measure of fat that must be eaten, we're going to see that the present diet works oppositely. Indeed, this eating regimen was made to quit eating an excessive number of fats, since it could prompt coronary illness, diabetes or elevated cholesterol. Furthermore, the maker, Nathan Pritikin, was determined to have a coronary illness, which brought about the formation of this eating routine. At his passing, during the examination, no indication of coronary illness was found. One needs to get that, in contrast to the fat flush eating regimen plans or the Bulletproof espresso diet, you have to realize that so as to have a sound way of life and heart, the ideal dinner plan doesn't exist without anyone else. Rather than searching for the ideal menu, you should concentrate on executing diet and activities.

## What is Pritikin Diet?

The Pritikin diet is known to be one of the healthiest diets ever created, and more than 100 studies have been done. The studies all agree on the fact that this diet is perfect for your body, and can prevent heart diseases, hypertension, and diabetes. But most importantly, this diet can help you lose weight.

The diet is based on a meager amount of fatty food options: there are about 10% of the calories taken in that come from fat sources. This diet allows you to eat a lot of whole grains and dietary fiber that are low in cholesterol and very low in fats.

There are two versions of this diet as they reworked the system to make it healthier and simpler. It is recommended to eat low calories food that provides a lot of bulk like carrots, broccoli, and dried beans. This way, the dieters can feel full and eat one's fill without having too many calories in their body.

The diet does not restrict you to the number of fruits and vegetables you can eat. It has much as you want, but it is recommended to eat little, and have 5 or 6 meals every day. So this diet is perfect for anyone who wants to lose weight and even better for people that wants to lower their fat.

As said at the beginning, it is known to be one of the healthiest diets in the world. And the reputation isn't based on nothing. There is a diet book for this diet and even a center where people go for a few weeks, and follow the diet. And when they come out, they're like new. This diet works, and Pritikin said that with this diet, your weight loss would be inevitable. You would lose weight step by step, but you would lose weight.

This diet is also known to be more than a simple menu. It's a lifestyle change, because of what you eat, and because of how you eat your life changes too. You feel better, healthier, and most importantly, you live better and longer.

It is recommended while you do this diet, to have some exercise every day. About 30-40 minutes of walking, running or working out, but exercising allows you to burn the fat faster.

## The pritikin diet plan

First of all, this diet doesn't claim that you will lose a certain amount of weight in any given amount of time. Instead, it's just proven that you will lose weight as long as you follow the guidelines of the diet.

And let's see how this diet works. What you can eat and what you can't, what you should do and what you shouldn't. It's not an obligation. It's just a way to make it work.

In this diet, the fruits, and vegetables will be your main food. But not only. You can eat a lot of whole grains food such as whole-wheat bread, whole-wheat pasta, brown rice, and oatmeal. This diet allows also eating starchy vegetables like corn, or potatoes.

The beans will also become one of your main food as you can eat all of them, black beans, red beans, pinto beans, garbanzo beans, all of them are good for you. But also peas and lentils. You'll also be able to eat lean calcium-rich food like nonfat dairy milk, nonfat yogurt, and fortified soymilk.

Fish will also be critical to add as it contains a great supply of omega 3-fatty acids. In the low amount of meat that you'll be able to eat, because you will have to eat some lean sources of protein, the skinless white poultry, the lean red meat like bison or venison are one of the few types of meat you can have.

Talking about proteins, some plants sources of protein like legumes or edamame (soybeans) are right for you. As you can see, the Pritikin diet works because it focuses on a vast diversity of whole (unprocessed) and minimally processed food.

Now let's have a look at all the food that won't be allowed in this diet. But one of the distinct things about this diet is that some foods are not especially good for this diet; but still, you can have some from times to times.

The less you eat of these tricky options, the better it is. But, you can still sometimes have some. We're talking about the oils, in general: these are not your best option on this system, but if you have to, you can have some of it, all the refined sweeteners like sugar, corn syrup or honey.

The less salt you eat, the better it is. But, if you need to season your plate, a small amount of salt can be tolerated. Also, you are expected to lower your intake of refined grains such as white pasta, white bread or white rice. Such options can be allowed but in their whole-wheat form. For the pasta, the bread, and the brown rice, you shouldn't have to eat a lot of them.

But what you can't eat in this diet, because it will make it less effective, are:

• All the saturated-fat-rich foods, like butter, tropical oils like coconut oil, cheese, cream, milk, and fatty meals.

• The organ meats: what you need to know when on this diet is that none of it is good for you.

• The same goes for the processed meat like hot dogs, bologna or bacon.

• And finally, you won't be able to eat the eggs yolks.

All of these foods increase the chance of weight gain and the risk of heart diseases, obesity, as well as numerous health concerns. If you are a person who likes to follow celebrities' way of life, you can check the Emily Ratajkowski diet.

About the beverages, water is always good for you, but so is non-processed cocoa if it's only up to 2 spoons a day. Caffeinated drinks are allowed too, and the same goes for alcoholic beverages. But, it always has to be taken in moderation.

All others drinks should be avoided. You may also take a look at the shibboleth diet phase 1.

Food Choices for a Lifetime Of Good Health

GO | Recommended Foods

5 or more servings daily of whole grains (such as whole wheat, oats, rye, brown rice, barley, quinoa, and millet); starchy vegetables (like potatoes, yams, and winter squashes); chestnuts; and legumes (beans, peas, and lentils). A serving is 1/2 cup cooked. For whole-grain bread products (like breads, bagels, and crackers), a serving is 1 ounce, which is generally half a common portion.

Limit refined grains (like white bread, white rice, and white pasta) as much as possible. But keep in mind that "white" does not necessarily mean "unhealthy." There are many healthy foods that are white, such as cauliflower, white potatoes, jicama, and nonfat yogurt.

Vegetables

5 (preferably more) servings daily. A serving is 1 cup raw or 1/2 cup cooked. Enjoy a variety of colors, like dark green, yellow, red, and orange vegetables. The more vegetables and other low-calorie-dense foods you eat, the less need there is for counting calories. You'll just naturally eat fewer calories, and shed excess weight.

Fruit

4 or more servings of whole fruits daily. For most fruits, a serving fits in your hand. Examples include all fresh and raw fruits, and frozen and canned fruits without added sugar. Enjoy whole fruit, not fruit juices. And don't believe silly science that says fruit is fattening.  To the contrary! People have shed 100 pounds and more with Pritikin's fruit-rich diet.

## Dairy and/or Dairy Substitutes

2 servings daily of dairy foods and/or dairy substitutes.

For dairy foods, choose from nonfat milk (1 cup), nonfat yogurt (3/4 cup), and nonfat varieties of ricotta and cottage cheese (1/2 cup). Choose plain nonfat milk, not flavored varieties like chocolate. Nonfat Lactaid is also acceptable.

For dairy milk substitutes, choose those that closely match the nutritional richness of nonfat cow's milk for calcium, vitamins D and B-12, and protein. Optimal choices tend to be fortified soymilks (original or unsweetened). Almond and rice milks usually score well for calcium, D, and B-12, but poorly for protein. So if you drink a cup of almond or rice milk, add to your daily diet a lean, protein-rich food like 1/2 cup cooked legumes (beans) or 2 egg whites. Steer clear of coconut milk because it contains saturated fat.

For all dairy milk substitutes, make sure they contain very little or no added sugars, sodium, and saturated fat.

Note: Many plant foods are rich sources of calcium, such as leafy greens like collard greens, turnip greens and kale, as well as tofu and tempeh.

Protein-Rich Foods

The healthiest diet on earth includes protein from both animal and plant sources.

Pritikin, one of the healthiest diets on earth, includes protein from both animal and plant sources.

Protein-Rich Animal Foods:

Fish, white poultry, lean meat

No more than 1 serving per day. A serving is about 3½ to 4 ounces cooked (the size of a deck of cards).

Below are fish/poultry/meat choices rated from "Best" to "Poor":

• Best: Omega-3-rich fish (such as salmon, sardines, herring, mackerel, and trout). Choose at least 2 times weekly. If you're using canned fish, such as canned sardines, select very-low-sodium or no-salt-added varieties.

• Good: Most other fish, plus shelled mollusks (clams, oysters, mussels, scallops).

• Satisfactory: Crustaceans (shrimp, crab, lobster),

• Poultry (white meat, skinless),

• Game meat (bison, venison, elk), optimally free-range and grass-fed.

• Poor: Red meat (beef, pork, veal, lamb, goat). For all red meat choices, select cuts that are under 30% fat.

For optimal heart-health results, limit "Satisfactory" choices to no more than 1 serving per week and "Poor" choices to no more than 1 serving per month.

Egg whites

Up to 2 daily. If you prefer egg whites instead of other land-based animal foods like white poultry and lean meat, you may eat more. About 7 egg whites is the protein equivalent of 1 serving of poultry or meat.  Steer clear of egg yolks and their high dietary cholesterol.

## Protein-Rich Plant Foods:

Legumes like beans, peas, and lentils

Soy products like tofu and edamame

For maximum cholesterol reduction and giving you the best chance at reversing atherosclerosis (heart disease), choose on most days protein-rich plant foods like beans instead of land-based animal foods like poultry and meat.  And yes, you can get plenty of protein with a plant-based diet.

## Healthiest Beverages on Earth

The healthiest diets on earth often include a bounty of fresh herbs in addition to whole, fiber-rich foods.

Water (plain, bottled, low-sodium, mineral); hot grain beverages (coffee substitutes); non-medicinal herbal teas (such as peppermint, rosehips, and chamomile); and cocoa – up to 2 tablespoons per day (use non-alkali processed cocoa). You do not have to drink large amounts of water daily. Simply drink when thirsty.

## Caffeinated Beverages

If you choose to drink caffeinated beverages, we recommend green or black tea over coffee because of tea's many health benefits. We also recommend moderation: no more than 400 mg of caffeine daily (the amount in about 4 eight-ounce cups of coffee or 8 eight-ounce cups of tea).

Coffee, both regular and decaf, does contain chemicals (diterpenes) that may modestly raise LDL cholesterol. However, by brewing with paper filters like paper cones or capsule filters like Keurig, the diterpenes are largely eliminated.

Alcoholic Beverages

Use in moderation or not at all.  For women, up to 4 drinks per week, with no more than 1/2 to 1 drink per day.  For men, up to 7 drinks per week, with no more than 1 to 2 drinks per day.  A drink is approximately 5 oz of wine, 12 oz of beer, or 1½ oz of 80 proof liquor.  Choose red wine over white wine, wine over beer, and either over liquor.


Herbs

Culinary herbs are rich sources of many beneficial phytonutrients, and are a good way to add flavor without extra calories, fat, or salt. Include at least 1 to 2 teaspoons of dried herbs or 1 to 2 tablespoons of fresh herbs each day.


## IF YOU WANT TO LOSE WEIGHT

Go wild on vegetables. The more vegetables, including dark green, yellow, red, or orange vegetables, the better! They're among the best foods for weight loss.

Limit calorie-dense foods such as dried grains (breads, crackers, cold cereals), dried fruits, nuts, and seeds. Avoid refined or concentrated sweeteners. They all pack a lot of calories into very small amounts of food. You'll find it much easier to feel full and satisfied and curb hunger if you focus instead on high-water, high-fiber foods like cooked grains (such as oatmeal and brown rice), vegetables, and whole fruits. These foods are low in calorie density.  You'll eat more – and weigh less.

Steer clear of fruit and vegetable juices because they provide less satiety than whole fruits and vegetables.


## IF YOUR WEIGHT IS FINE

Celebrate! Eat as many whole grains, vegetables, legumes (such as beans and peas), and fruits as you want. Enjoy more calorie-dense foods such as avocados and nuts, but limit them to keep your weight under control. Limit avocado intake to no more than 2 ounces per day. Limit walnuts, flaxseeds, almonds, pumpkin seeds, pecans, pistachios, sunflower seeds, filberts (hazelnuts), peanuts, cashews, and macadamia nuts to no more than 1 ounce per day.


Refined Fats & Oils

Limit the consumption of ALL oils to no more than 1 teaspoon per 1000 calories consumed, especially if you're trying to lose weight, because oils have the highest calorie density of any food or ingredient.

Refined or Concentrated Sweeteners

For healthy individuals who choose to use sweeteners, a suggested rule of thumb is a maximum of 2 tablespoons of fruit juice concentrate or 1 tablespoon of other refined sweeteners (such as barley malt, corn syrup, rice syrup) per 1000 calories consumed. None is optimal. Avoid fructose and high fructose corn syrup.

Salt and High-Sodium Foods, Condiments

Avoid added salt, and highly salted, pickled, and smoked foods. Limit foods that have more than 1 mg of sodium per calorie so as not to exceed 1200 to 1500 mg of sodium per day, depending on age. It's one of the most important things you can do to lower blood pressure.

Refined Grains

Limit as much as possible foods containing refined grains (such as white pasta, white bread, and white rice).

# RECIPES

Salsa Chicken

Here's the easiest recipe ever! It's just two ingredients: chicken breasts and salsa. (Do read labels to make sure you're getting low-sodium or no-salt-added varieties of salsa.)

You simply put a pound or two of boneless, skinless chicken breasts on the bottom of the crockpot. Then pour salsa over the top of the chicken, enough to cover the chicken about one-half inch.

Then turn on the crockpot. You're done!

If you're new to slow cooking, do read the user manual so that you're aware of any requirements regarding your particular crockpot.

For Salsa Chicken using my crockpot, I simply set the temperature to LOW. In four hours the chicken breasts are nicely cooked.  I then remove the lid and with a fork shred the breasts so that the salsa soaks in everywhere.

I put the lid back on and let the shredded chicken sit there in the nice warm crockpot for a few minutes, heat turned off, while I get the rest of dinner ready.

What emerges from the crockpot is a deliciously juicy chicken that can be used in all sorts of ways.

Make fajitas by ladling some of your chicken into whole-wheat tortillas with sliced green bell peppers and onions, stir-fried or raw.

Use your Salsa Chicken as a topping over a big green salad (you don't even need salad dressing) laced with sliced radishes and cucumbers, or any crunchy-style veggies you have on hand.

Ladle your chicken over a cooked whole grain like brown rice. It works really well as a potato topper, too.

Or whip up a super easy Mexican-style soup by adding your Salsa Chicken to a pot on the stove with some low-sodium chicken broth, pinto beans (canned, no salt-added), and corn (just pour in a cup or so from a bag of frozen corn). Heat your soup for about 15 minutes, and enjoy.


## Lentil and Barley Soup

Want the deep, slow-cooked flavors of rich, creamy beans and barley without spending a lot of time in the kitchen? Try our delicious crockpot Lentil and Barley Soup.

Servings  Prep Time Cook Time

62-cup portions 20minutes 6hours

Ingredients

7 cups vegetable broth (low sodium)

1 can tomatoes diced, (14.5 ounces, no-salt-added, undrained)

1.5 cups lentils (dry) rinsed

1 cup onions chopped

1 cup carrots chopped

1 cup celery chopped

1 cup mushrooms sliced

3/4 cup barley uncooked

5 cloves garlic minced

1 tablespoon Italian Seasoning (salt-free)

1 teaspoon thyme (dried)

3/4 teaspoon black pepper

Servings:

6

 2-cup portions Units:

Course Main Dish, Soup, Vegetarian

Cuisine American, Easy, Vegan, Vegetarian

Instructions

Combine all ingredients in a 4-quart or larger crockpot. Cover. Cook on HIGH setting 5 to 6 hours or until lentils are desired tenderness. If using LOW setting, cook 10 to 12 hours or until lentils are desired tenderness.

Setting the heat

The cooking temperature for crockpots is the same on all settings – about 210 degrees. So the setting you choose (usually LOW or HIGH) merely dictates how quickly your slow cooker gets to that temperature.

I like using the LOW setting as often as I can because I find that its slower, gentler cooking does a really nice job of bringing out flavors. And with 8-plus hours of cooking time, I can be gone all day from the house and not worry about dinner overcooking.

One more note: Most modern slow cookers will automatically convert to a "warming" setting at the end of cooking. So if you're getting home a little later than expected, you know dinner isn't overcooking.


Prepping the night before

There's no need to get up early in the morning to chop up ingredients for your evening's crockpot dinner.

Instead, prepare everything the night before. Put your ingredients into your slow-cooker's ceramic pot, and cover and store in the refrigerator overnight. Come morning, get it out, lower it back down into your slow cooker machine, turn it on, and walk out the door.

## Converting recipes

For converting recipes you already have into crockpot-style cooking, here are some general guidelines:

If a dish usually takes 1 to 2 hours on the stove, cook it in your crockpot for 3 to 4 hours on HIGH or 6 to 8 hours on LOW.

If a dish usually take 2 to 4 hours on the stove, cook it in your crockpot for 4 to 6 hours on HIGH or 8 to 12 hours on LOW.

Root vegetables such as beets, carrots, onions, parsnips, potatoes, radishes, and turnips can take longer than other vegetables, so put them near the heat source – the bottom of the pot.

Here's our third healthy crockpot recipe. It takes just a few minutes to assemble but delivers loads of hearty, snappy flavor.

## Cajun-Style Red Beans and Rice

Our Cajun-Style Red Beans and Rice takes just a few minutes to assemble but delivers loads of hearty, snappy flavor.

Servings  Prep Time Cook Time

6one-cup servings 20minutes 7hours

Ingredients

2 cups red kidney beans (dried) rinsed

1 cup brown rice uncooked

1  red onion chopped

1  green bell pepper chopped

4 stalks celery chopped

6 to 8 cloves garlic minced

1/2 cup chives finely chopped

4 teaspoons Cajun seasoning (salt-free)

1 tablespoon paprika (smoked)

5 cups water

Servings:

6

 one-cup servings Units:

Course Dinner, Main Course, Side Dish

Cuisine Easy, Mexican, Vegan, Vegetarian

Instructions

Add all your ingredients to your crockpot, veggies on top. Cook on LOW for around 7 hours. Cooking times may vary depending on your crockpot.

Wing it!

As Chef Anthony and his fellow chefs at the Pritikin Longevity Center have always taught, don't constrain yourself with written recipes.


Go with what you like any ingredients you like! Some experiments may not first turn out as well as you imagined, but that's okay. Make notes. Incorporate them the next time. When it comes to cooking any kind of cooking practice makes perfect.

• Put your dried beans, root vegetables, and seasonings on the bottom of your crockpot.

• Add enough stock or water to cover your ingredients about one-quarter to one-half inch.

• Then add your other veggies – a nice hefty pound or two.

• Turn on your crockpot. Then walk away!


## One Pan Mexican Quinoa

Ingredients

1 Avocado

1 (15-ounce) can Black beans

2 tbsp Cilantro, fresh leaves

1 cup Corn, canned or roasted frozen kernels

2 cloves Garlic

1 Jalapeno

1 Lime, Juice of

1 (14.5 oz) can Tomatoes, fire-roasted

Canned Goods

1 cup Vegetable broth

Pasta & Grains

1 cup Quinoa

Baking & Spices

1 tsp Chili powder

1 Kosher salt and freshly ground black pepper

Oils & Vinegars

1 tbsp Olive oil

Nuts & Seeds

1/2 tsp Cumin


The Cilantro & Lime Infused Quinoa with Black Beans

Ingredients :

3/4 cup of black beans dry,

½ of onion sliced, one jalapeno sliced,

Three cloves of garlic,

Two sliced and

One clove only minced, bunch cilantro leaves minced,

a cup  of tomatoes diced, with the seeds removed,

1/2 cup of onion chopped,

1/4 cup of jalapenos diced,

seeds removed for a milder flavor.

Rinse the black beans and soak them during the night. Rinse the black beans once again and place them in a medium pot with two cups of water, and a half sliced onion, one sliced jalapeno, and three cloves of sliced garlic. Bring it to a boil, then reduce heat to stew and cook until it's soft, so for about 40 minutes. The yield is about two cups of cooked black beans. Now put the rinsed Quinoa and one 1/4 cups of water in a medium pot. Make it boil, then cover, reduce heat to medium-low, and stew until the water is absorbed about 15 minutes. Stir into juice and zest from two limes and a quarter cup of chopped cilantro. Cover for 5-6 minutes. In a medium bowl, mix one cup of diced tomatoes, half a cup of diced onion, a quarter cup of diced jalapenos, one clove of minced garlic, one handful of chopped cilantro, and juice and zest from 1 lime. Layer the beans, Quinoa, and salsa on a plate, and it's ready.

## Oatmeal chocolate chip cookies

Cookies cups ounces unbleached all-purpose flour½ teaspoon baking powder¼ teaspoon freshly grated nutmeg½ teaspoon Tablespoons 2 sticks unsalted butter, softened but still cup packed ounces light brown

Blueberry Quinoa Parfait

25 minutes

Blueberry Quinoa Parfait Recipe : Quinoa used in a breakfast parfait layered with vanilla yogurt, fresh blueberries and toasted pecans.

Ingredients

Produce

2 cups Blueberries

Pasta & Grains

1 cup Quinoa

Dairy

2 cups Vanilla yogurt

Liquids

2 cups Water

Other

1/4 cup Pecans, toasted and coarsly chopped


Vegetarian Chili

Slow but oh-so-good cooking. That's what this vegetarian chili's all about. Want to add leftover shredded roasted chicken or turkey breast? Go right ahead. Poultry- or veggie-style, it's a wonderful one-pot dish for chilly winter evenings or party nights in front of the T.V.

Servings  Prep Time Cook Time

12half-cup servings 30minutes 70minutes

Ingredients

1/4 cup green bell pepper diced

1 cup red onion diced

1/2 cup garlic chopped

1 cup So Soya ground. See Recipe notes.

2 tablespoons All Purpose Seasoning See Recipe notes.

1  chipotle pepper

1/2 cup corn kernels (fresh or frozen)

3 cups red beans cooked, (If using canned varieties, purchase no-salt-added.)

1/4 cup shallots chopped

1 teaspoon oregano , dry

3 tablespoons thyme (fresh) leaves picked and chopped

1 teaspoon chili powder

1 tablespoon balsamic vinegar

1 cup tomato puree no-salt-added

1/2 cup carrots medium-diced

1 cup tomatoes diced

1 quart vegetable stock (low-sodium)

1 tablespoon Veggie Grated Topping, Parmesan Flavor See Recipe notes.

1/4 cup cilantro leaves chopped

Servings:

12

 half-cup servings Units:

Course Lunch, Main Dish, Side Dish, Soup/Stew, Vegetarian

Cuisine American, Comfort Food, International, Vegetarian

Instructions

• In a large nonstick stockpot, sauté bell peppers, onion, and garlic at medium-high heat until brown, about 3 minutes.

• Meanwhile, soak So Soya in ½ cup hot water for about 5 minutes. Drain excess liquid. Add So-Soya and All Purpose Seasoning to stockpot, and cook for 3 minutes.

• Add remaining ingredients, except Veggie Grated Topping and cilantro, and simmer for 1 hour.

• Finish off with Veggie Grated Topping and freshly chopped cilantro. Remove chipotle pepper before serving.

• Serve with whole-wheat, low-sodium pita chips, brown rice, mashed potatoes, or simply by itself.

## Recipe Notes

So Soya is a dehydrated soybean product. It is available in some supermarkets nationwide as well as online at sosoyafoods.com.

Make your own All Purpose Seasoning by blending granulated onion, granulated garlic, salt-free lemon pepper, and paprika.

Strawberry Yogurt Swirl

Ingredients

Vegetarian, Gluten free

· Makes 10

Produce

1 cup Blueberry

1/2 cup Raspberries

1 cup Strawberry

Condiments

1 tbsp Splenda

Baking & Spices

1 tsp Vanilla extract

Dairy

2 cups Yogurt, fat free


## Creamy Celery and Asparagus Soup

In warm weather, try this soup chilled, suggests Chef Anthony. And once again, have some fun. Play with ingredients. Love garlic? Add more! Like fresh oregano and have some sitting in the fridge? Add it! Enjoy Quinoa? Use quinoa instead of brown rice.

Ingredients

Vegetarian

· Serves 12

Produce

1 cup Asparagus spears

2 tbsp Basil, fresh

4 cups Celery

4 tsp Garlic

1 cup Onion

1 tbsp Thyme, fresh

1 cup Yellow tomato

Canned Goods

8 cups Vegetable broth, no-salt-added

Condiments

2 tsp Soy sauce, low sodium

Pasta & Grains

1 cup Brown rice, cooked

Baking & Spices

1 pinch Peppercorns, black ground

1 pinch Pritikin seasoning

# Spinach Marmalade Chicken

Servings

4people

Ingredients

4 4-ounce chicken breasts (boneless, skinless) butterflied

1 tablespoon fresh garlic mince

1 teaspoon stoneground mustard (sodium-free)

1 pound fresh spinach chopped

2 tablespoon orange marmalade (100% fruit)

1 cup fresh pineapple peeled and pureed

1/4 cup white wine

Instructions

• Preheat oven to 350 degrees.

• Rub chicken breasts with garlic and mustard.

• Combine spinach and marmalade. Spoon mixture over inner side of each breast.

• Roll each breast. Place breasts on nonstick baking sheet, and bake at 375 degrees until done, about 20 minutes.

• Meanwhile, in a skillet stove on medium heat, combine pineapple and wine, and reduce until thickened, about 5 minutes.

• When chicken breasts have finished cooking, slice each one into 3 to 4 slices and serve on pineapple/wine sauce.

• Slice chicken breast. Serve on sauce.

## Crustless Butternut Cheesecake

This Crustless Butternut Cheesecake has zero saturated fat and only about one-tenth the calories of regular cheesecake, but loads of creamy, dreamy flavor.

Ingredients

Vegetarian, Gluten free

· Serves 12

Refrigerated

1/2 cup Egg whites

1 package Silken tofu

Condiments

1/2 cup Splenda

Baking & Spices

2 tbsp Vanilla

Dairy

4 oz Cottage cheese, low-sodium fat-free

1 lb Cream cheese, fat-free


## Witch's Potion Pie

1.5 hours

Did you know that a slice of traditional pumpkin pie often has 5 grams of artery-crippling saturated fat? It's like eating a cheeseburger for dessert! And really, who needs it when you can enjoy deeply satisfying pumpkin flavor with Pritikin Chef Anthony Stewart's zero-saturated-fat pie.

Ingredients

Vegetarian

· Makes 8

Produce

1/2 Butternut s<uash, large

1 Garnish 8 blackberries

1 Garnish blackberry puree

8 Party favor pumpkins

2 cups Pumpkin

Refrigerated

3 Egg whites

1/2 cup Soymilk

Breakfast Foods

2 cups Corn flakes

Condiments

1 tsp Lime juice

1/4 cup Splenda

Baking & Spices

1/4 tsp Cardamom, powder

1 tsp Cinnamon, powder

3 tbsp Vanilla extract

## Chicken Veggie Burgers

1 lb skinless chicken breast ¼ cup chopped onion ¼ cup chopped celery ¼ cup chopped carrot 1 tsp chopped garlic 1 tsp Pritikin All-Purpose Seasoning In a food processor, chop chicken till ground on med-high heat, sauté veggies till translucent-3 minutes. In a large mixing bowl, combine ground chicken, vegetables, and seasoning. Mix until fully incorporated. Mold mixture into 8 4 oz patties On a hot nonstick skillet, sear patties on each side to your desired doneness.

## Banana Ricotta Ice Cream

Servings Prep Time

6 ` 15minutes

Ingredients

1 pound bananas (very ripe) peeled, vacuum sealed, and frozen

1 cup ricotta cheese (fat-free)

2 tablespoons orange juice

1 teaspoon orange zest

¼ teaspoon nutmeg ground

1 teaspoon vanilla extract

Servings:

6

 Units:

Course Dessert, Entertaining

Cuisine Easy, Quick, Vegetarian

Instructions

• Remove bananas from freezer and let sit for 5 minutes (until they begin to defrost around the edges).

• Place ricotta cheese in a food processor and pulse.

• Chop the bananas and add to the food processor along with all remaining ingredients. Puree until smooth and creamy.

• Scoop mixture into a plastic bowl and cover with food-grade plastic wrap, making sure the plastic wrap touches the top of the mixture. Place in the freezer for 15 to 20 minutes.

• Scoop or pipe into individual serving bowls or parfait glasses.

- Recipe Notes

- If desired, garnish with a raspberry and a sprig of rosemary. Another healthy delight for a hot season!

## Roasted Corn Salad

From the chefs at the Pritikin Longevity Center in New Dehli, India, comes this zesty, no-salt-added Roasted Corn Salad. Easy to make. Enjoy it all through corn-on-the-cob season.

Servings Prep Time Cook Time

4people 30minutes 10 minutes

Ingredients

3 to 4 ears sweet corn on the cob (Your goal is 2 cups of corn kernels after they have been sliced from cobs).

1  white onion sliced

2  green bell peppers (or green capsicum peppers), sliced

2  tomatoes sliced

DRESSING

1 tablespoon lemon juice

2 pinches  red chili powder

1 teaspoon cumin powder

Servings:

4

 people Units:

Course Dinner, Entertaining, Vegetarian

Cuisine Easy, Indian, Vegan, Vegetarian

Instructions

• For dressing, combine three ingredients. Mix well.

• For remaining ingredients: Remove stalk/green leaves from corn cobs. Roast corn cobs directly over grill flame until corn is slightly roasted on all sides. Using a sharp knife, remove corn kernels from cobs. Discard cobs.

• In a large bowl, combine corn kernels, onion, green peppers, and tomatoes.

• Pour dressing on top. Toss well. Serve immediately.

## Very Berry Ice Cream

Servings Prep Time

8  10minutes

Ingredients

2  bananas

1 cup  strawberries (frozen)

1 cup blueberries (frozen)

1 cup raspberries (frozen)

Up to 1/2 cup  soymilk

1/4 cup apple juice concentrate (frozen)

Servings:

8

 Units:

Course Dessert, Entertaining, Vegetarian

Cuisine Easy, Quick, Vegan, Vegetarian

Instructions

• Four to six hours prior to dessert time, peel and slice bananas. Seal in plastic bag and place in freezer.

• Just before serving, put frozen berries and bananas in a food processor. Pulse fruit and add soymilk to desired creamy consistency. Add apple juice concentrate. Blend.

• Freeze what you don't eat tonight in individual servings for future desserts.


Strawberry Souffle

50 minutes

No butter, cream, sugar, or anything else that hurts your heart and health in this strawberry souffle. Just a lovely, airy strawberry-sweet dessert!

Ingredients

Vegetarian, Gluten free

Produce

4 pints Strawberries

Refrigerated

4 Egg whites

1 lb Tofu silken, firm

Condiments

2 Tablepoons splenda

Baking & Spices

1 tsp Vanilla extract

## Mashed Potatoes with Corn and Fat-Free Sour Cream

45 minutes

Oh, the rewards of easy, healthy cooking! Here's a creamy, comfort-food-style creation - Mashed Potatoes with Corn and Fat-Free Cream.

Ingredients

Vegetarian, Gluten free

· Serves 8

Produce

1 cup Corn

2 lbs Potatoes

Baking & Spices

1 Dash Nutmeg

Dairy

1/2 cup Milk, very hot nonfat

1/4 cup Sour cream, fat free

## Grilled Pineapple

Grilled Pineapple recipe from ifood. This very simple sweet dessert is the perfect ending to a heavy barbecue. The pepper brings out the grilled

Ingredients

Gluten free

· Makes 4

Produce

1/2 tsp Garlic, granulated

1 Jalapeno pepper, fine

1 Pineapple

Canned Goods

2 tbsp Apple juice concentrate

Condiments

1 tsp Soy sauce

Baking & Spices

1/4 tsp Black pepper

1/4 tsp Chili powder

1/2 tsp Cinnamon


## Vegetable Quesadilla

This recipe is by a guest favorite at the Pritikin Center. Pritikin Cooking School Chef, Ernesto Alonso Aguila.

Ingredients

Produce

2 tbsp Cilantro

Condiments

1/4 cup Pico de gallo

Bread & Baked Goods

2 Tortilla, Whole-wheat

Dairy

4 tbsp Mozzarella cheese, fat-free

4 tbsp Sour cream, fat free

Other

4 cup Vegetables (sliced thin and suteed)

## Healthy Deviled Eggs - No Yoke!

The typical filling for deviled eggs is loaded with the artery-clogging fats in egg yoke and mayonnaise. Pritikin Executive Chef Vincent Della Polla keeps all of the classic flavors of deviled eggs, but replaces the egg yolks and mayonnaise with...wait. You'll never guess!

Ingredients

1 Quart egg whites

4 ounces cream cheese, fat free

1 tablespoon tumeric (mixed with hot water to make a thin paste)

2 tablespoon chives chopped

1 tablespoon dill

1 tablespoon Dijon mustard (low-sodium)

1 tablespoon stoneground mustard (no-salt-added)

1 teaspoon paprika (garnish)

Servings:

4

 Units:

Cuisine American

Instructions

• Spray small casserole pan with cooking spray and pour in egg whites.

• Cover with aluminum foil and bake for 20 minutes or until egg is firm at 350F

• Remove foil and allow egg to completely cool down.

• Use a small round cookie cutter to make circular egg white shapes.

• Use a melon baller and remove a small part from the center of each egg round.

• Take the leftover egg in the pan and whip it in the food processor with remaining ingredients.

• Use a pastry tip and bag to pipe the egg mixture onto each egg round.

• Garnish with sprinkled paprika and chives.


## Braised Orange Ginger Sea Bass

We're wild over Chef Vincenzo Della Polla's new seafood menu. Try this effortlessly elegant dish with your favorite veggies and steamed brown rice.

Servings Prep Time Cook Time

4  4Minutes 6Minutes

Ingredients

4 4 ounce Sea Bass

1 teaspoon Pritikin All-Purpose Seasoning

1 teaspoon Pritikin Shake it Seasoning

3 oranges Zest & Juice

2 teaspoons ginger sliced

25 cup apple juice

25 cup apple cider vinegar

5 cup white wine

Servings:

4

Units:

Cuisine American, Asian, Easy, Fish

Main Dish Fish & Seafood

Instructions

• Mix dry spices together and coat Sea Bass.

• In a hot skillet sear fish for 2 minutes.

• Add remaining ingredients and cover.

• Lower heat and cook over low heat for 4 minutes.

Get tons of nutritional goodness plus tons of delish with these Sweet Potato Pancakes With Blueberries.

Servings

124 oz. pancakes

Ingredients

2 medium sweet potatoes

3 cups skim milk

1 cup egg beaters

1 teaspoon vanilla extract

2 cups whole wheat flour

2 teaspoons baking powder

2 teaspoons baking soda

1 teaspoon cinnamon ground

3 tablespoons Splenda

Light spray  Pam

1 pint blueberries fresh

Servings:

12

 4 oz. pancakes Units:

Course Breakfast, Vegetarian

Cuisine American

Instructions

• Preheat oven to 400 °F.

• Wash potatoes and pat dry. Poke several times with a fork. Wrap each potato in foil. Place on middle oven rack. Place a baking sheet on rack below potatoes to catch any drippings of natural sugars. Bake until very soft to the touch, about 50 to 60 minutes. (Potatoes can be cooked days in advance.)

• Allow potatoes to cool. Then remove skin.

• In a large mixing bowl, blend potatoes with skim milk, egg beaters, and vanilla extract.

• In a separate large mixing bowl, combine all dry ingredients (whole wheat flour through Splenda), and mix well.

• Make a well in the center of the dry mixture bowl. Pour the potato mixture into the center. Using a wire whip, whisk until smooth, using a circular motion.

• Preheat nonstick omelet pan or griddle on medium flame. Lightly spray with Pam.

• Use an ice cream scoop to portion each pancake onto preheated pan or griddle. Sprinkle blueberries on top of each cake.

• Cook for 2 minutes. Flip. Cook another 2 minutes.

Recipe Notes

These Sweet Potato Pancakes with Blueberries are especially yummy when served with Pritikin Creamy Vanilla Sauce.


## Beet & Mango Salad

Servings

1people

Ingredients

1 pound red beets peeled and cooked

1 pound carrots peeled, diced and steamed

1 cup mango ripe, peeled and diced

1/2 cup blueberries

4 cup mixed greens lettuce

1/4 cup Pritikin Outrageous Asian Salad Dressing or Pritikin Tuscan Sunshine Italian Salad Dressing

Servings:

1

 people Units:

Course Appetizer, Main Course, Main Dish, Salad, Side Dish

Cuisine American, Vegan, Vegetarian

Instructions

• On a bed of mixed greens arrange equal amounts of beets, carrot, blueberries and mango.

• Drizzle with Pritikin Outrageous Asian or Pritikin Tuscan Sunshine Italian Salad Dressing.


## Apple Mango Salsa

Ingredients

fresh mangoes chopped

fresh apple chopped

red onion chopped

red pepper chopped

fresh cilantro and parsley chopped

fresh lemon juice

fresh lime juice

Servings:

4

Units:

Course Sauce, Vegetarian

Cuisine American, International, Vegan, Vegetarian

Instructions

• Combine all ingredients together in bowl and mix well.

• Store in refrigerator before serving.

Instead of using heavy mayonnaise and white potatoes, opt for fat-free sour cream and sweet potatoes, which are a great source of potassium, dietary fiber and many vitamins. With the added diced apples, this salad is the perfect balance of hearty, crunchy and sweet.

Ingredients

5 cup sweet potatoes diced

2 cup apples diced

1 tablespoon lemon juice

8 ounces sour cream, fat free

1/2 tablespoon cinnamon

1 tablespoon apple juice contentrate (frozen

1/2 tablespoon vanilla extract

1 pineapple Heat oven to 400 degrees. (as you like) chunks

1 strawberries (if you desire, as gains) diced

Servings:

4

Units:

Course Salad

Cuisine American, International, Vegetarian

Instructions

• Heat oven to 400 degrees.

• Slice and dice sweet potatoes in desired size and shape.

• Bake in oven for 30-40 minutes, until soft and slightly crisped.

• Allow sweet potatoes to cool.

• Add apples and sweet potatoes to a large salad bowl.

• In a small bowl, combine lemon juice, sour cream, cinnamon, apple juice concentrate and vanilla extract. Mix well.

• Pour over apples and sweet potatoes and combine ingredients well.

• Refrigerate for 30 minutes before serving.

• Garnish with pineapple chunks and sliced strawberries if desired.

## Beet and Potato Puree

Want something fabulously flavorful and colorful for a side dish? And veggie-rich to boot? Try our Pritikin chefs' Beet and Potato Puree. Doll it up, if you're in a Martha Stewart mood, by placing each serving in a heart-shaped mold.

Servings Prep Time Cook Time

4  20minutes 20 minutes

Ingredients

1 pound red beets peeled and chopped

1/2 pound russet potatoes peeled and chopped

1/2 medium onion chopped

1 teaspoon garlic chopped

1 pint water

Servings:

4

 Units:

Course Side Dish, Vegetarian

Cuisine American, Easy

Instructions

• In a large pot, combine all ingredients and bring to a boil. Reduce heat and simmer until beets and potatoes are tender, about 20 minutes.

• Drain, removing all liquid. Puree beet/potato mixture in a food processor or by mashing with a wire whip.

## Vegan Butternut Cheesecake

This Crustless Butternut Cheesecake has zero saturated fat and only about one-tenth the calories of regular cheesecake, but loads of creamy, dreamy flavor.

Ingredients

2 tablespoon apple juice concentrate

1 package Silken Tofu (12.3oz)

1/4 cup Roasted Butternut squash pureed

2 tablespoon Splenda

2 tablespoon vanilla

1 teaspoon cream of tartar

1 teaspoon xanthan gum

Servings:

4

 Units:

Course Dessert

Cuisine American, International, Vegan, Vegetarian

Instructions

• In a food processor combine all ingredients and puree until smooth.

• Pour into individual muffin cups or pie dish

• Bake at 375 degrees for 30 minutes in a hot water bath.

## Spicy Seafood Soup

This Spicy Seafood Soup is always a hit in the dining room at the Pritikin Longevity Center. Cook up a big batch on the weekend and enjoy all week long. You can freeze this soup, too.

Servings  Prep Time Cook Time

8 to 101-cup servings 35minutes 3-1/2hours

Ingredients

1 pound shrimp shells call your fish market in advance to set aside shells for you.

1 gallon water

1 carrot diced

1 onion Vidalia, diced

3 stalks celery diced

1 fennel bulb cored, diced

1/2 cup okra diced

2 tablespoons garlic chopped

1/4 cup tomato puree no salt added

1 bay leaf

3 tablespoons thyme fresh, chopped

1 chipotle pepper whole

1 teaspoon oregano dry

1/2 pound scallops diced

1 pound white fish diced (good choices: halibut, sea bass or tilapia)

1 tablespoon Pritikin Fish Seasoning or any salt-free fish seasoning

1 teaspoon crushed red pepper flakes

1/2 pound shrimp diced

1 cup whole baby clams, low sodium

  black peppercorns freshly ground, to taste

1/2 bunch fresh cilantro leaves chopped

Servings:

8

 1-cup servings Units:

Course Dinner, Lunch, Soup

Cuisine Fish, Fusion, Gourmet

Main Dish Fish & Seafood


Instructions

• For your stock, simmer shrimp shells (feel free to add carrot peels, celery leaves, fennel greens, and onion skins) in 1 gallon water for 2 hours. Strain and reserve stock.

• In a large stockpot, add carrots, onions, celery, fennel, and okra, and cook on medium-low heat until onions are translucent, about 5 minutes.

• Add shrimp stock, garlic, tomato puree, bay leaf, thyme, chipotle, and oregano. Simmer for 2 hours.

• Add scallops, white fish, Pritikin Fish Seasoning, and red pepper flakes, and simmer for 1 hour more, breaking fish with back of spoon.

• In last 5 to 10 minutes of cooking, add shrimp, clams, and black pepper. Simmer till shrimp and clams are cooked. Remove chipotle and bay leaf. Garnish with cilantro. Serve.

Recipe Notes

Pritikin Fish Seasoning can be purchased at the online Pritikin Market.

## Spaghetti Squash and Tomato Salad

When paired with tomato and basil, spaghetti squash is a darn good replacement for spaghetti. Think of it as faux-pasta.

Servings  Prep Time Cook Time

2 cupsper serving 5minutes 25minutes

Ingredients

2 spaghetti squash cut in half lengthwise and seeds removed

1 cup tomatoes diced

1/2 cup basil fresh and chiffonade

1/2 cup Pritikin Outrageous Asian Salad Dressing available online.

Servings:

2

 per serving Units:

Course Main Dish, Salad, Side Dish, Vegetarian

Cuisine Comfort Food, Quick

Instructions

- Pre-heat oven to 400 degrees.

- Place spaghetti squash cut side down on a baking tray and bake until soft (usually about 25 minutes).

- Use a spoon to scoop out the inside of the squash and cool.

- Toss diced tomatoes with basil and combine with squash and Outrageous Asian Salad Dressing .

- Toss lightly and serve.

Recipe Notes

This dressing is great as a marinade as well.

Pritikin Outrageous Asian Salad Dressing is available online in the Pritikin Market.


## Chilled Raspberry and Cucumber Soup

Gourmet but so easy to whip up! This Chilled Raspberry and Cucumber Soup is an exquisite combination of rich berry flavor and refreshing cucumber. Plus, in your favorite soup bowls, it's pretty and bright.

Servings Prep Time Cook Time

8  10minutes 0minutes

Ingredients

3 cups raspberries fresh, rinsed

1 cup cucumber seedless variety, chopped

1/4 cup apple juice concentrate frozen (thawed), undiluted

3 cups water

1/4 cup cucumber seedless, finely diced for garnish

Servings:

8

 Units:

Course Entertaining, Soup, Vegetarian

Cuisine Easy, International, Quick

Instructions

• In a blender, combine all ingredients except finely diced cucumber. Blend.

• Chill. Serve garnished with finely diced cucumber on top

Recipe Notes

Chef's note: Fresh basil or mint goes nicely with this soup.

## Carrot-Stuffed Bison Tenderloin

Servings Prep Time Cook Time

8  20minutes 60minutes

Ingredients

Carrot Stuffed Bison Tenderloin

2 whole carrots peeled

2 tablespoons

2 tablespoons salt free lemon pepper

2 tablespoons ground coriander

2 pounds grass-fed bison tenderloin cleaned, ends removed

## Blueberry Balsamic Reduction

2 cups blueberries

1 cup balsamic vinegar

Servings:

8

Units:

Course Entertaining, Main Course

Cuisine American, Bison, Gourmet

Instructions

• Carrot Stuffed Bison Tenderloin

• Place a roasting pan in the oven at 400 degrees to pre-heat.

• Blanche carrots: Put them, whole, into a pot of boiling water for 5 minutes, then immediately throw them into a bowl of ice water. Remove them after 5 minutes, and pat them dry with a paper towel.

• In a small bowl, combine all-purpose seasoning, lemon pepper seasoning, and coriander. Rub mixture all over tenderloin.

• Insert a boning knife, lengthwise, into the center of tenderloin. Then turn, making a hole. Repeat from the other end.

• Insert the whole carrots into the center incisions, making sure that the carrots meet in the center.

• Lower oven heat to 250 degrees. Roast tenderloin until medium-rare (our Pritikin chefs' recommendation for the best flavor), which is until a meat thermometer reads 135 degrees (usually about 1 hour). Allow the tenderloin to rest on the carving board for 15 minutes before slicing.

• Blueberry Balsamic Reduction

• While tenderloin is finishing up in the oven, combine In a sauce pan on the stove the blueberries and balsamic vinegar. Bring to a boil.

• Reduce flame and let simmer for 10 minutes. Cool and blend in a food processor. Serve with bison.

Recipe Notes

* You can purchase Pritikin's salt-free All-Purpose Seasoning online at the Pritikin Store. Or make your own all-purpose seasoning by blending together your favorite herbs and spices such as paprika, garlic powder, onion powder, dried oregano, and dried basil.

Drizzle this Chambord Raspberry Coulis over just about any dessert, from fruit to Pritikin Cheesecake, that would pair well with its deep raspberry tones. This a sauce that makes everything it graces more beautiful and luscious.

Prep Time Cook Time

3minutes 0minutes

Ingredients

1 cup raspberries (fresh) rinsed

1 tablespoon Splenda

2 tablespoons Chambord Liqueur

Servings:

4

 Units:

Course Dessert, Entertaining, Sauce

Cuisine Easy, Quick

Instructions

• Combine ingredients in a blender. Blend until smooth.

• Chill and serve.

Recipe Notes

Goes nicely with dessert or fresh fruits.


## Chicken in Sweet Chili Sauce

Servings

4oz

Ingredients

4 4ounces chicken breast skinless

1 tablespoon

1/4 cup whole wheat flour (optional)

3 tablespoon sweet chilli pepper (crushed)

1/4 cup apple juice (concentrated) (or 2 tablespoons of splenda)

1 cup hot water

1 teaspoon corn starch

Servings:

4

oz Units:

Course Lunch, Main Course, Main Dish

Cuisine Poultry

Instructions

• Season chicken breast with all purpose seasoning

• Combine sweet chili pepper, hot water and apple juice concentrate and let sit for 10 minutes.

• Lightly flour chicken breast and sear in a medium hot skillet on both sides

• Pour sweet chili mixture over chicken and cover. Lower flame and turn chicken on other side and cook for 8 minutes.

• Mix cornstarch with 2 tablespoons cold water and thicken.

Recipe Notes

Chef's note: add garlic, onion and any herb you like for a more delicious dish.

## Thai-Style Vegetable Stir Fry

Servings Prep Time Cook Time

4people 30minutes 10minutes

Ingredients

1 tablespoon garlic chopped

1 tablespoon ginger root peeled and chopped

1/4 cup 100% frozen apple juice concentrate thawed, undiluted

2 tablespoons Dijon mustard, no-salt-added

1/4 cup vegetable stock (low-sodium)

1 zucchini sliced into thin strips

1 red bell pepper sliced into thin strips

1 Vidalia onion sliced into thin strips

1 head broccoli stems and florets chopped

1/2 pound button mushrooms wiped clean, sliced in half

1/4 bunch cilantro leaves chopped

2 tablespoons cornstarch

2 tablespoons water

Servings:

4

people Units:

Course Dinner, Entertaining, Vegetarian

## Cuisine Asian, Easy

Instructions

• In a wok or nonstick skillet, sauté garlic and ginger until glossy.

• Add apple juice, mustard, and half of vegetable stock, stirring to combine.

• Add remaining ingredients (except cornstarch and water). Sauté for 5 minutes.

• Whisk cornstarch in water, and add to thicken stir fry.

## Pritikin Caesar Salad

Servings Prep Time Cook Time

2 to 4people 20minutes 0minutes

Ingredients

1 box tofu (lite silken)

1/4 cup lemon juice

3/4 tablespoon Angostura Worcestershire sauce

2 tablespoons Dijon mustard, no-salt-added

2 cups white balsamic vinegar

2 tablespoons garlic minced

1 tablespoon 100% apple juice concentrate (found in freezer sections) thawed, undiluted

2 ounces water

4 cups chopped Romaine lettuce

1 teaspoon Parmesan cheese fat-free

Servings:

2

 people Units:

Course Lunch, Salad

Cuisine American

Instructions

• In a food processor or blender, combine all ingredients except Romaine and Parmesan.

• Process until dressing is completely smooth and creamy.

• Combine desired amount of dressing with Romaine and Parmesan.

• Refrigerate remaining dressing.

## Bread Pudding

Servings

8

Ingredients

4 cups whole wheat bread (low-sodium) cut into cubes

1/4 cup Splenda

2.5 cups soy milk or skim milk

1 teaspoon cinnamon

2 tablespoons raisins

1/2 teaspoons nutmeg

1 teaspoon vanilla

3 egg whites

Servings:

8

Units:

Course Dessert, Entertaining, Vegetarian

Cuisine American, International, Vegetarian

Instructions

• Soak bread in milk and add spices

• Fold in egg whites

• Bake at 350 for 25 minutes.


Chili with "ground beef"

Ingredients

1/4 cup bell pepper diced

1 cup ground so-soya soaked in 1/2 cup hot water

1 cup onion (red) diced

1/2 cup garlic chopped

3 tablespoons Green Grotto

1/2 cup corn kernels

3 cups red beans cooked

2 tablespoons Pritikin A.P. spice mix (no salt)

2 teaspoons oregano

1 teaspoon basil

1 teaspoon chilli powder

2 teaspoons paprika

1/3 bottle enrico mild salsa

1 tablespoon balsamic vinegar

1/2 tomato puree (no salt)

1 cup veggie juice (no-salt added)

1/2 cup carrots medium diced

1/2 cup tomato diced

1/4 teaspoon liquid smoke

Servings:

4

Units:

Course Dinner, Dip, Lunch, Main Course, Main Dish, Side Dish, Soup/Stew, Vegetarian

Cuisine American, Vegan, Vegetarian

Instructions

• Cook Red beans until just soft in 3 cups water.

• In a separate stockpot sauté peppers, onion & garlic until brown.

• Add So-Soya and no salt spice mix and cook for 3 minutes

• Add all ingredients except veggie topping and cilantro and simmer for 1 hour.

• Serve with whole wheat pita chips, brown rice, mashed potato or by itself


## Stuffed Mushrooms

Ingredients

15 large mushrooms (white buttom)

1 box tofu (silken)

5 tablespoons pita bread crumbs (whole-wheat)

1/2 teaspoons garlic

1 tablespoons parsley chopped

1/2 teaspoon Grey Poupon mustard (low-sodium)

1 bushel spinach fresh

1 tablespoon onion chopped

2 tablespoon red bell pepper chopped

Servings:

4

Units:

Course Dinner, Lunch, Main Course, Main Dish, Vegetarian

Cuisine American, International, Vegan, Vegetarian

Instructions

• Take cap off mushrooms.

• Saute, onion, pepper and garlic until brown.

• Add spinach and let wilt down

• Blend vegetable mix in the food processor

• Mash tofu and add to the rest of ingredients, mix well.

- Fill mushroom top with half tablespoon of mixture.

- Bake at 350 degrees for 30 minutes.


## Strawberry Mousse

Servings

10

Ingredients

2 pounds tofu (firm silken)

2 cups strawberry puree cooked

2 tablespoons vanilla extract

1/4 cup Splenda

 rasberries as garnish

Servings:

10

 Units:

Course Dessert, Entertaining, Vegetarian

Cuisine American, International, Italian, Vegan, Vegetarian

Instructions

• Puree tofu in food processor until very smooth.

• Add remaining ingredients. Puree until thoroughly combined and fluffy.

• Put into serving glasses.

• Garnish each serving with a raspberry.


## Seafood Ceviche

Ingredients

1 pound shrimp peeled and deveined

1 onion (red) thinly julienne

1/2 teaspoon garlic finely chopped

1 jalapeno pepper chopped

1/2 bushel cilantro chopped

1 bushel parsley chopped

1/4 cup lemon juiced and zest

2 bell peppers julienne

Servings:

4

 Units:

Course Dinner, Dip, Lunch, Main Course, Main Dish, Side Dish

Cuisine American, International, Latin American, South American

Main Dish Fish & Seafood

Instructions

• In a plastic or wooden bowl combine all ingredients and mix well.

• Let stand in the refrigerator over night

• Serve in an iceberg lettuce cup or over mixed greens

## Seared Salmon

Servings

4portions of 4oz

Ingredients

3 bell pepper julienne

2 carrot julienne

1 red onion julienne

1 teaspoon garlic minced

1 pound salmon cut into 4oz portions

1 tablespoon

Servings:

4

portions of 4oz Units:

Course Dinner, Lunch, Main Course, Main Dish

Cuisine American, Continental

Instructions

• Coat salmon in spice.

• In a hot skillet, brown salmon.

• Cover, cook until cooked though.

• Time depends on the thickness of the fish.

• In a separate pan, brown vegetables then add garlic at the end.



## Crispy Breaded Cauliflower

Try other vegetables like zucchini or broccoli. Try other seasonings like lemon pepper, garlic powder, onion powder

Ingredients

1 head cauliflower broken into smaller pieces

1/4 cup whole wheat flour

3 tablespoon egg whites or egg beaters

1/2 cup whole wheat whole grain bread crumbs

1 tablespoon

Servings: 4

Units:

Course Appetizer, Lunch, Side Dish, Snack, Vegetarian

Cuisine American, International, Vegetarian

Instructions

• Preheat oven to 400 F

• Cut cauliflower and steam for 2-3 minutes, cooking it only partially.

• Take some whole grain bread and grind into bread crumbs in the food processor.

• Season the flour and bread crumbs.

• Dip cauliflower in flour, then into the egg, then into the bread crumbs.

• Spray a sheet tray with cooking spray

• Place cauliflower on tray and bake for 30-45 minutes or until desired crispiness.


## Seared Bison with Spinach, Mushrooms & Balsamic

Servings

4portions of 4oz

Ingredients

1 pound bison cut into 4oz portions

1 tablespoon

1 pound mushrooms (assorted)

10 ounces fresh spinach sliced

4 tablespoons balsamic vinegar

 pint grape tomatoes

Servings:

4

 portions of 4oz Units:

Course Dinner, Lunch, Main Course, Main Dish

Cuisine American

Instructions

• Toss tomatoes in dry basil, oregano, garlic and balsamic.

• Roast tomatoes for 30 minutes at 400F

• Coat bison in spice.

• In a hot skillet brown bison & mushrooms.

• Cover & turn heat to low, cook for 5 minutes

• Add spinach & tomatoes. Cover for 2 minutes more.

• Serve immediately



## Seared Chicken with Sauté Julienne Vegetables

Servings

4

Ingredients

3 bell peppers

2 carrots

1 onion

1 zucchini

4 4oz portions CHICKEN

1/4 teaspoon basil

1/4 teaspoon granulated onion

1/4 teaspoon granulated garlic

1/4 teaspoon chili powder

1/4 teaspoon coriander ground

1/4 teaspoon black peppercorns ground

1 tablespoon paprika

Servings: 4

Units:

Course Dinner, Lunch, Main Course, Main Dish

Cuisine American, International, Poultry

Instructions

• Coat chicken in spice. I

• In a hot skillet brown chicken with no oil or water.

• Cover cook until cooked though.

• Time depends on the thickness of the chicken.

## Spicy Pickled Vegetables

Ingredients

3 bell pepper julienne

2 carrot julienne

1 red onion julienne

1 teaspoon garlic minced

1 teaspoon red pepper crushed

1 teaspoon oregano dried

1 tablespoon red wine vinegar

2 teaspoons apple juice concentrate

1 tablespoon

Servings: 4

Units:

Course Side Dish, Vegetarian

Cuisine American, Continental, Vegetarian

Instructions

- In a hot pan, brown vegetables then add garlic halfway thru.

- Deglaze with liquids and add seasoning.

- Let reduce for 2 minutes. Serve on top of seared fish.

## Hodgson Mill Vegan Spiral Pasta with Vegetables

Servings Prep Time Cook Time

8people 10 minutes 12minutes

Ingredients

16 ounces spiral pasta (whole wheat non-GMO, Hodson Mill)

1 small tomatoes (organic)

1 medium rainbow carrot (organic)

1 cup broccoli (organic)

Dressing

1 tablespoon garlic powder (organic)

1 tablespoon onion powder (organic)

1 tablespoon Splenda

2 tablespoon oregano (dry & organic)

2 tablespoon black pepper

1/4 tablespoon thyme (dry & organic)

1 tablespoon parsley (dry & organic)

1/2 tablespoon pepper flakes (organic)

3/4 cup red wine vinegar

Servings: 8

people Units:

Course Dinner, Lunch, Main Course, Main Dish, Vegetarian

Cuisine American, International, Italian, Vegetarian

Instructions

• Cook the pasta according to the packages directions, then rinse with cool water until the pasta is cold.

• Add your chopped vegetables and dressing to the cold pasta, mix well and enjoy. This salad is even better the next day, so go ahead and make it ahead of time.


## Grilled Salmon with Watermelon and Fresh Mint Salsa

Servings Prep Time Cook Time

4people 10minutes 15minutes

Ingredients

1/8th watermelon seedless

1/2 yellow pepper

1/2 cucumber

1/2 lemon freshly squeezed

6-8 fresh mint leaves

4 salmon steaks

Servings: 4

people Units:

Course Dinner, Lunch, Main Course, Main Dish

Cuisine American, Fish, Fusion, International

Instructions

• Finely dice watermelon, pepper and cucumber.

• Chop and add mint, reserving a couple leaves for garnish.

• Squeeze in lemon juice and mix well.

• Grill salmon until cooked throughout (about 10 - 15 minutes)

• Let cool slightly and spoon salsa over fish.


## Cilantro Lime Roasted Chicken

Servings Prep Time Cook Time

8people 10minutes 50minutes

Ingredients

2 pounds chicken breasts (skinless)

2 tablespoons cilantro chopped

1 lime zested and juiced

1 tablespoon no-calorie sweetener sucralose (Splenda) or stevia

2 cloves garlic minced

1/2 teaspoon black pepper freshly ground

Servings: 8

 people Units:

Course Dinner, Entertaining, Lunch, Main Course, Main Dish

Cuisine Easy, International, Poultry

Instructions

• Preheat oven to 375 degrees F.

• Arrange the chicken breasts in a single layer in a nonstick baking pan.

• In a small bowl, whisk together the cilantro, lime zest, lime juice, no-calorie sweetener, garlic, and black pepper. Pour the mixture evenly over the chicken.

• Bake until the internal temperature of the largest piece of chicken is 165 degrees, about 45 to 50 minutes.

Servings Prep Time Cook Time

4people 15minutes 25minutes

Ingredients

4 pieces salmon fillet

1 bunch kale fresh

2 tomatoes

1 yellow pepper

1/2 red onion

4 cloves garlic

1 carrot

1/2 teaspoon powdered turmeric

1/2 teaspoon cumin powder

1 teaspoon lemon juice

1/2 teaspoon black pepper

1/2 teaspoon red pepper flakes crushed

Servings: 4

People Units:

Course Dinner, Lunch, Main Course, Main Dish

Cuisine Fish

Instructions

• Place salmon fillets in a pan, drizzle lemon juice on top, sprinkle black pepper, 1/4 tsp. turmeric and 1/4 tsp. cumin. Bake at 400 for about 15 minutes

• Rinse vegetables thoroughly then slice them up. Use a vegetable peeler to thinly slice the carrot into ribbons

• Mince garlic cloves and place them in a wok with a few teaspoons of water. Then add kale, red pepper flakes, 1/4 tsp. cumin and 1/4 tsp. turmeric, cover and steam for 6 minutes

• Remove salmon from oven and shred with a fork

• Add onions, yellow pepper, red onions, carrots, tomatoes and shredded salmon to wok. Stir on medium heat for about 6 minutes

## CONCLUSION

The consequences of this diet, dissimilar to the McDougall diet food list, are as of now demonstrated since many individuals go to Pritikin focuses to help shed pounds and decrease their danger of heart illnesses. Keep in mind, this framework is not the same as other eating regimen plans.

This eating regimen is known to decrease up to 23% the all-out cholesterol, diminish by 33% the Triglycerides, yet additionally lessen the constant irritation, bring down the insulin level by 46% and mitigate the metabolic conditions to all individuals doing this eating routine, regardless of how old they are. Yet additionally bring down the dangers of malignant growths and diminish the speed of disease cells development. At the point when you follow this routine, you won't need to consider other diets supplements.